THE COMPLETE GUIDE TO THE BEST INTERNATIONAL FISH MAIN COURSES

The Complete Guide to International Cookbooks on the tastiest fish dishes, a must-have collection for all fish lovers.

By Author

Antonino Top Chef

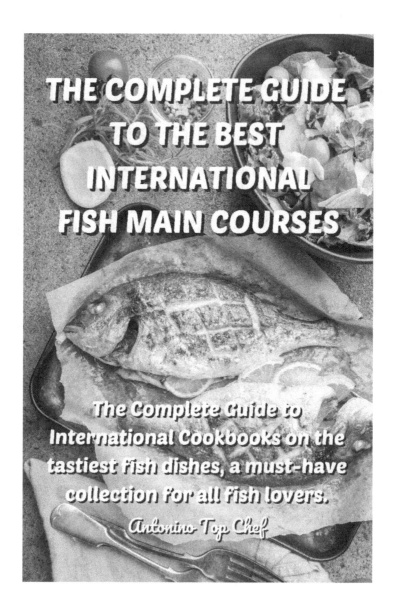

THE COMPLETE GUIDE
TO THE BEST
INTERNATIONAL
FISH MAIN COURSES

The Complete Guide to
International Cookbooks on the
tastiest fish dishes, a must-have
collection for all fish lovers.

Antonino Top Chef

Table Of Contents

☆ 55% OFF for BookStore NOW at $ 24,95 instead of $ 35,95! ☆

If you are looking for and love to eat fish, in this guide you will find everything you need to cook fantastic dishes and amaze your fellow travelers.

Have fun and cook with love

START IS NOW!!

Buy is NOW and let your Customers get addicted to this amazing book!

Lemon herb hake fillet with garlic tomatoes

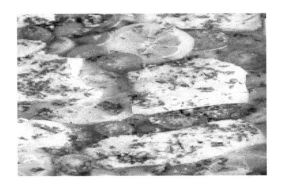

Ingredients

- Russet potatoes (1½), cut into quarter ijmchr
- ¼ cup of extra virgin oil
- Three garlic cloves.
- Salt and pepper to taste
- Four skinless bake fillers
- An inches thick if four sprigs
- Fresh time
- A lemon sliced thin.

Preparation

Heat oven to 426 degrees. In a bowl toss potatoes with two Tablespoons of oil, add salt and pepper. Heat it without viberekng, stir in the microwave. Take the potatoes from the microwave into a baking dish (13 by 9inch). Line the side skinned on potatoes. Drill the Jake with two Tablespoons of olive oil. Add sprigs, fbhme on top. Bake till you can easily part it when prodded. Serve.

Nutritional value

- Carbohydrate 19g
- Fat 23
- Protein 27g
- Fiber 5.7

Pan roasted halibut with chermoula

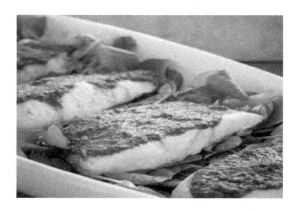

Ingredients
- Fresh cilantro leaves (¾)
- Olive oil (¼)
- Tablespoons of olive oil(¼)
- Tablespoons of lemon juice(2)
- Four garlic minced cloves
- Half teaspoons of ground cumin
- Half teaspoon of paprika
- Salt (¼) teaspoon.
- Cayeene peooer fish(⅛)
- Two (1¼-pound) skin-on full halibut steaks,
- One to one and half inches thick and 10 to 12 inches long,
- Salt and pepper and pepoer to taste.
- Olive oil (2 Tablespoons)

- ✓ For The Chermoula
  Blend all ingredients in the food processor til smooth, for one minutes. Reserve for serving.
- ✓ For The Fish
  Heat up the oven, season the halibut placed on a paper towel with salt and pepper. Make the oil not then fry in a non stick skillet for a high heat till it's smokimg. Cook halibut I'm kt for five minutes.
- ✓ Flip a bit the halibut, use spatula to to that, then put in a different skillet

With caution move the halibut to the board, lose the aluminum foil, allow to rest for five minutes. Take skin away from.the steaks, separate meat from.bones
Serve it with chermoula.

Pan roasted Monkfish with oregano black olive relish

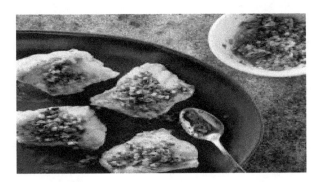

Ingredients

- Olive oil (¼)
- Two Tablespoons of minced oregano
- Two Tablespoons of red wine vinegar
- One small shallot
- A teaspoon of Dijon
- Salt and pepper to taste.
- Pitted Kalamata olives (¼)
- Four minced skinless monkfish fillers.
- One to one and half inches thick
- Half teaspoon of sugar

Preparation

Microwave two Tablespoons if oil wut oregano in a small bowl. Allow mixture to mix thoroughly. Beat shallot, vinegar, mustard and a quarter teaspoon of pepper. Add olives in, keep aside for serving. Cooke wraopoed monkfisj, add salt and pepper, then sugar. Heat up Tablespoons of oil in a twelve imce ovensafe pan. Cook till it turns brown for about two minutes. Flip with spatula. Move the skillet to I've, roast the monkfish for eight to twelve minutes. Serve relisb

Grilled whole sardines

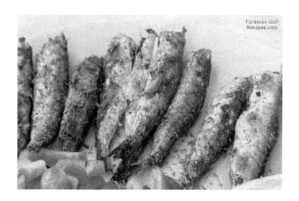

Ingredients

- Twelve whole sardines, prepare it for coomk g
- Two tablespoons of mayonnaise.
- Half teaspoon of honey
- Lemon wedges.

Preparation

Wash over running water. Season with pepper the captivity. Add honey and mayonnaise in it. Cook on charcoal grill or gas. Clean the garage, brush grate with oil till it's black. Cook over the grill till it's skim is brown. Flip the sardines with soatual, keep coomjng, add lemon wedges to serve.

Pan roasted sea bass

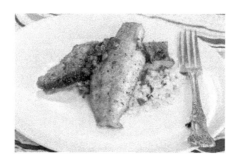

Ingredients

- Four - skinless sea bass fillets,
- One to one and half inches thick
- Salt and pepper to taste
- Half teaspoon sugar
- 1 tablespoon extra-virgin olive oil
- Lemon wedges

Preparation

Cook over heat of 426, degrees. Pat dry with oaoae towels, add salt and pepper to season. Sprinkle sugar on it. Gcook on a heated oil placed on medium high heat for two minutes. Keep flipping the sides. Roast till the too it can easily give way while cutting with knife.

Pan-Roasted Sea Bass with Green Olive, Almond, and orange

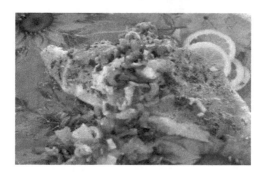

Ingredients

- Half cup of silvered almonds
- Half cup of pitted brine cured green olives
- One small garlic cloves,
- A teaspoon of grated orange
- Blend everything in a food processor,
- Put in bowl and put the orange juice, police oil, fresh mint and two teaspoon of white wine vinegar. Use salt to season and cayenne to tast
- Serve with fish.

Pan-Roasted Sea Bass with Roasted Red Pepper,Hazelnut, and Thyme Relish

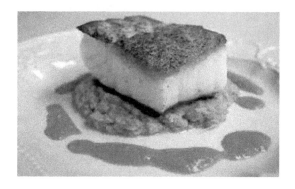

Ingredients

- Half cup of toasted and skimmed hazelnuts
- Half cup of jarred roasted pepper
- One mince garlic cloves
- Half teaspoon of lemon zest

Preparation

Blend everything together in a food processor. Trssnfer to the bowl, stri olive oil, two Tablespoon of fresh parsekt, four teaspoon of lemon juice, a teaspoon of mimved fresh time and quarter teaspoon of paprika. Add salt and pepper to taste. Serve with the fish.

Sauteed sale Fish

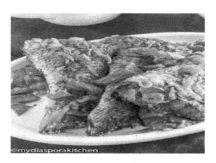

Ingredients

- Half cup of alll-purpose flour
- 8 skinless sole fillets, quarter - to half inch thick
- Salt and pepper to taste
- Quarter cup of olive oil
- Lemon wedges.

Preparation

Add salt and pepper to the flour in the shallow disb, oat the fish with it.

Fry in a pan, flip it with spatula. Transfer on a platter, losen the aluminum foil.

Serve with lemon wedges.

Sautéed Sole with Fresh Tomato Relish

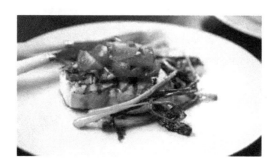

Ingredients and Preparation

Add two ripe tomatoes, seedee, cut it to quarter pieces, two chopped fresh basil, a tablespoon of olive oil, a small minved garlic cloves. A teaspoon of red wine vinegar in a bowl. Leave to for fifteen minutes add salt and paper. Serve with sole.

Sautéed Sole with Grapefruit and Basil Relish

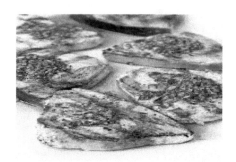

Ingredients and Preparation

Cut the peel away, cut the grapefruit into eight wedges, slice each into half inch. Out the grapefruit in a strainer, leave to drain for fifteen minutes. Keep a drained juice apart, add tkhwgr with fesh basil, minved shallot, two Tablespoons of lemon juice, two extra virgin oil. Add salt and pepper to taste. Serve with sole.

Grilled swordfish with Italian salsa verde

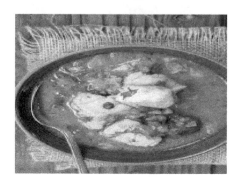

Ingredients and Preparation

Four skin on swordfish steaks, one to one and half inches. Two Tablespoons of olive oil. Add salt and pepper to taste. Half cup of Italian salsa verde. Dry with paper towel, add salt and pepper with oil. Grill over charcoal or gas grill. Brush the cooking grate consistent like five to ten times to make it glissg. Grill the swordfish for 6-9 minutes. Flip each sides gently. Use parking knife to prod to check if it's done. Serve with italian salsa verde.

Sicilian fish stew

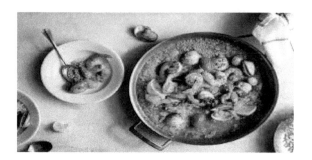

Ingredients

- Quarter cup of pine nuts
- Quarter cup of chopped fresh mint
- Four garlic cloves
- A mincee teaspoon
- Two tables of extra virgin oil
- Two onions
- One fine chopped celery rib, minced
- Salt and pepper
- A teaspoon.of fresh thyme
- One can of whole peeled tomatoes, drained with juice reserved, chopped ccoarseteo
- Two bottles clam juice ¼ cup golden raisins
- Two fblespoons capers, rinsed
- One and half pounds skinless swordfish steaks,
- One to one inches thick,

Preparation

Add pine nuts, mint, garlic, orange zest inside a bowl keep aside for serving Cook onions, celery, ½ teaspoon salt, and ¼ teaspoon pepper till it's soft, for five minutes. Cook tyme, pepper flakes, and remaining garlic till fragrant for thirty seconds. Steam wine and tomato juice. Cook for four minutes, with tomatoes, clam juice, raisins, and capers, for fifteen minutes. Cook swordfish in pot, season usk g salt and pepper. Cook for three minutes. Add salt and pepper to season. Serve with pine nuts.

Clams with pearl couscous, chorizo and leaks

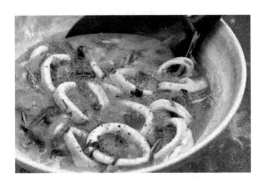

Ingredients

- Two cups pearl couscous
- Salt and pepper to taste
- Two tablespoons of extra-virgin olive oil
- One and halfpounds leeks, white and light green parts only,
- halved lengthwise, sliced thin, and washed well six ounces of chorizo sausage.
- A tablespoon of moved thyme.
- Frsh parsley

Preparation

Boil water in a pan. Pour cousocus, St and cook till firm for eight minutes. Pour leeks and chorizo into the oil with garlic, thyme, vermouth. Pour tomatoes in. Cook till valams open up for about eight to twelve minutes. Transfer clams into a big pot. Throw away anynoe that won't open up. Stir the couscous and parsley into cooking liquid and add salt and pepper to taste. Serve

Nutritional value

- Carbohydrate 13g
- Fat 15g
- Protein 32g

Calamari stew with garlic and tomatoe

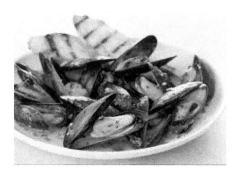

Ingredients

- Cup (¼) of olive oil, extra for serving 2 onions,
- Chopped two celery ribs
- Eight gaic cloves sliced.
- Red pepper flakes (¼)
- (½) cup of white whine
- Salt and pepper
- Three can of whole peeled tomatoes
- Pitted green leaves (⅓)
- A tablespoon of capers
- Three Tablespoons of minced fresh parsley.

Preparation

Cook in the heated oil celery, galric and poeor for thritu seconds, pit wine in, and cool till it's almost evaporated for one minute. Add Salt and pepper to squid. Stir in pot; allow steaming for fifteen minutes. Pour tomatoes, olives, capers I'm till is soft for about 30-35 minutes. After it's done stir parsley, season with salt and pepper to taste.
Serve

Oven steamed mussels

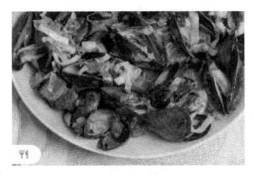

Ingredients

- Three Tablespoons of olive oil
- Three garlic cloves, move the red pepper flakes
- Four pounds of mussel, scrubbed
- Teaspoon of salt (debeared)
- Two tablespoons of fresh parsley.

Preparation

Heat up the oven to 495 degree. Pour a tablespoon of oil, garlic, and pepper flakes in large roasting pan on top.of the pot. Cook, keep stiring til it's fragrant for thirty seconds. Pour wine in, thyme, sprigs, bay leaves, boil, cook till wine has reduced a bit. Cook mussel to most have opened. Take out the mussels after 18 minutes. Throw the ones that refuse to open away. Add two Tablespoons of oil to It and serve.

Nutritional value

- Carbohydrate 4g
- Protein 17g
- Fat 9g

Seared scallops with orange lime dressing

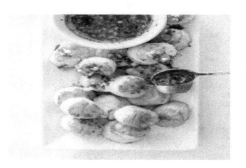

Ingredients

- One and half pounds large sea scallops, tendons removed
- Six tablespoons extra-virgin olive oil
- Two tablespoons orange juice
- Two tablespoons lime juice
- One small shallot, minced
- One tablespoon minced fresh cilantro
- Teaspoon red pepper flakes (⅛)
- Salt and pepper to taste.

Ingredients

Put your scallops in baking sheet layered within kitchen towels that are clesn.put the second towel on top of scallops. Press it lightly to allow liquid blots. Leave to sit for some time for about 10 minute. Beat half cup oil, orange juice, lime juice, shallot, cilantro, and pepper flakes into a bowl. Add Salt to season. Cook in a heated skillet, till it becomes brown. Turn both sides. Once it's done move to a serving plate, loose foil. Add scallops to serve.

Garlicky roasted shrimp with parsley and anise

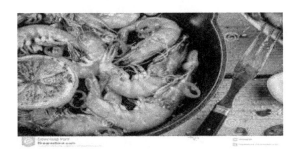

Ingredients

- Quarter cup salt
- Two pounds shell-on jumbo shrimp (16 to 20 per poindd
- Half quarter cup extra-virgin olive oil 6
- garlic cloves, minced 1 teaspoon anise seeds
- Half teaspoon red pepper flakes quarter
- teaspoon pepper
- Two tablespoons minced fresh parsley Lemon wedges

Preparation

Put salt in 4 cups of cold water in a big container and dissolve use sharp kitchen chairs used to cut the shell of shrimp but make sure you don't remove the shell used a knife to keep cutting the shrimp into half inch deep put shrimp in Bryan cover it up and put in freezer for 15 minutes mix oil garlic pepper flakes pepper and anise seeds in a big bowl Paul your shrimp parsley and oil then flip it well ensure that the oil get into the innermost part of a shrimp lime shrimp in a single layer on a rock and put in a baking sheet. Boy your shrimp till it becomes opagei, and when the shelves are turning brown do this for about 4 minutes flip on its side rotate every 2 minutes then serve with your lemon wedges

Nutritional value

- Carbohydrate 7g
- Fat 4g
- Protein 16g

Shrimp and white beans

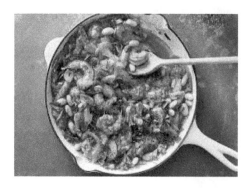

Ingredients

- A pound extra-large shrimp peeled and deveined Pinch sugar
- Salt and peppe
- Five tablespoons extra-virgin olive oil
- A red bell pepper, stemmed, seeded, and chopped fine
- 1 small red onion, chopped fine
- Two garlic cloves, minced
- Quarter cup of aspoon red pepper flakes
- Gsk (15-ounce) cans cannellini beans, rinsed
- Two xjps baby arugula, chopped
- Coarse 2 tablespoons lemon juice

Preparation

Dry shrimp with the Welsh people add sugar salt and pepper to season. Heat a tablespoon of oil in a non sticky skillet on top of high heat until it starts smoking then add shrimps to the skillet and cook do not stay cook till Easter spotting Brown cook for about 1 minute take it off it toss the shrimp let it sit for about 30 seconds then move the shrimp to a bowl and cover to keep it warm heat up the remaining quarter cup of oil in a in an empty skillet include bell pepper onion and half teaspoon of salt and cook till it gets soft for about 5 minutes but in your pepper flakes and garlic and cook until fragrant for about 30 seconds but your beans in and cook until the it passes through it for 5 minutes finally pour hrimp and arugula weeds any of the juices keep flipping till the irregular is wilted for 1 minute then pour in lemon juice and season with salt and serve your meal.

Nutritional value

Carbohydrate 8g
Protein 23g
Fat 1g

Mink fish tagine

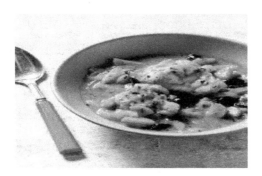

Ingredients

- Three (2-inch) strips orange zest 5 garlic cloves, minced
- Two ablespoons extra-virgin olive oil 1 large onion, halved and sliced ¼ inch thick 3
- carrots, peeled, halved lengthwise, and sliced ¼ inch thick Salt and pepper
- A tablespoon tomato paste 1¼ teaspoons paprika
- A teaspoon ground cumin
- Half teaspoon dried mint
- Quarter teaspoon saffron threads,
- crumbled 1 (8-ounce) bottle clam juice
- 1½ pounds skinless monkfish fillets,
- One to one and half inches thick, trimmed and cut into 3-inch pieces ¼
- Cup pitted oil-cured black olives,
- Quartered 2 tablespoons
- Minced fresh mint 1

- Teaspoon sherry vinegar.

Preparation
Cut a strip of orange zest mix with a teaspoon garlic in bowl; reserve. Cook the ingredients in the pot till they are light brown for 10-20 mounted. Pour the remaining garlic, tomato paste, paprika, cumin, dried mint, and saffron and cook till fragrant, for 30 seconds. Cook fish, steam it for 12miutes. Stir in olives, fresh mint, vinegar, and garlic–orange zest mixture. Season with salt and pepper to taste. Serve.

Nutritional value
- Carbohydrate 16g
- Fat 3g
- Protein 28g

Bouillabaisse

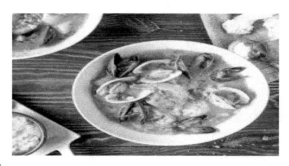

Ingredients

- Quarter cup of olive oil
- A small fennel bulb, stalks discarded, bulb halved, cored, and chopped fine 1 onion,
- chopped fine
- Eight garlic cloves, minced
- A teaspoon minced fresh thyme or ¼ teaspoon dried ¼ teaspoon saffron threads,
- crumbled ⅛ teaspoon red pepper flakes ¾ cup dry white wine or dry vermouth
- Two (bottles clam juive)

Preparation

Cook feneml, onion till it'ssodt for five minutes. Add garlic, thyme, oeoee flakes and saffron. Cook till it's fragrant. Stir in the wine, cook till the water is reduced a bit. Stir in the clam juice, tomatoes with their juice, and bay leaves. Steam it. Cook halibut for two minutes. Arrange shrimps over the stew, cover it and keep cooking till it flakes apart of you prod it with knife. When the shrimps and scallops are firm and mussels is ooened. Serve in shallow bowls

Nutritional value

- Carbohydrate 27g
- Fat 7
- Protein 34g

Cioppino

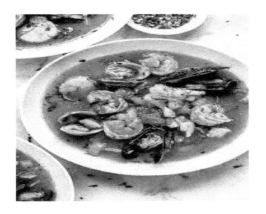

Serves 6
Ingredients - Allergies: SF, GF, DF, EF, NF

- 3/4 cup coconut oil
- 2 onions, chopped
- 2 cloves garlic, minced
- 1 bunch fresh parsley, chopped
- Cups stewed tomatoes
- 1.5 cups chicken broth
- 2 bay leaves
- 1 tbsp. dried basil
- 1/2 tsp. dried thyme
- 1/2 tsp. dried oregano
- 1 cup water
- 1-1/2 cups white wine
- 1-1/2 pounds peeled and deveined large shrimp
- 1-1/2 pounds bay scallops
- 18 small clams

- 18 cleaned and debearded mussels
- 1-1/2 cups crabmeat
- 1-1/2 pounds cod fillets, cubed

Preparation

Over medium heat melt coconut oil in a large stockpot and add onions, parsley and garlic. Cook slowly, stirring occasionally until onions are soft. Add tomatoes to the pot. Add chicken broth, oregano, bay leaves, basil, thyme, water and wine. Mix well. Cover and simmer 30 minutes. Stir in the shrimp, scallops, clams, mussels and crabmeat. Stir in fish. Bring to boil. Lower heat, cover and simmer until clams open.

Crab Cakes

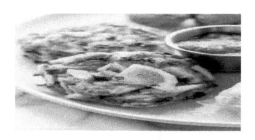

Ingredients

- 3 lbs. crabmeat
- 3 beaten eggs
- 3 cups flax seeds meal
- 3 tbsp. mustard
- Three tbsp. grated horseradish
- 1/2 cup coconut oil
- 1 tsp. lemon rind
- 3 tbsp. lemon juice
- 2 tbsp. parsley
- 1/2 tsp. cayenne pepper
- 2 tsp. fish sauce

Preparation

In medium bowl combine all ingredients except oil. Shape in to smallish hamburgers. In fry pan heat oil and cook patties for 3-4 minutes on each side or until golden brown. Optionally, bake them in the oven. Serve as appetizers or as main course with large fiber salad.

Nutritional value

- Carbohydrate 19g

- Fat 7g
- Protein 32g

Spicy Shrimp With Angel Hair Pasta

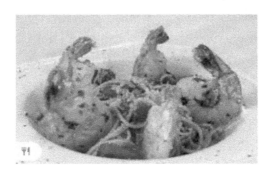

Ingredients

- Eight ounces angel hair pasta
- One and half of pounds medium shrimp, peeled and deveined
- A teaspoon low-calorie baking sweetener
- Quarter teaspoon salt
- A tablespoon chili powder
- Half teaspoon ground cumin
- ½ teaspoon ground coriander
- ½ teaspoon dried oregano
- 1 tablespoon + 1 teaspoon extra-virgin olive oil
- Lime wedges for garnish

Preparation

Bring water to a boil, add pasta, and cook pasta until al dente. Remove from heat, drain pasta, and return to pot, drizzling with scant amount of olive oil to keep pasta from sticking together. Set aside. Sprinkle shrimp with sweetener and salt. Combine chili powder, cumin, coriander, and oregano, then lightly coat shrimp with spice mixture. Heat 1 tablespoon of olive oil in a large nonstick over medium-high heat. Add half of the shrimp and sauté about 4 minutes, or until cooked. Remove cooked shrimp from pan and repeat procedure with 1 teaspoon olive oil and remaining shrimp. Divide cooked pasta into 4 servings, top with shrimp and pan sauce, and garnish with lime wedges. Serve immediately.

Italian Poached Scallops

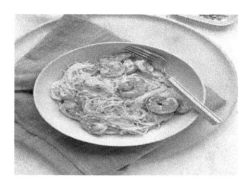

Ingredients

- A cup fresh orange juice
- A pound fresh sea scallops
- Two teaspoons grated orange peel
- A small ripe plum tomato, chopped
- A teaspoon chopped fresh marjoram
- Two tablespoons low-fat sour cream
- Salt and freshly ground pepper to taste

Preparation

In a big nonstick skillet over medium heat, bring orange juice to a boil. Reduce heat and add scallops and orange peel. Cover and simmer 5 minutes or until scallops are opaque and tender. Remove scallops from heat and transfer to a plate; cover to keep warm. Add tomato and marjoram to orange juice sauce and simmer for roughly 2 minutes until liquid reduces to half of original amount. Stir in sour cream and cook until sauce thickens. Add salt and pepper to taste. Return scallops to skillet, mix with sauce, and heat through. Serve immediately with risotto and/or vegetables. Approx. 148 calories per serving

Nutritional Value

- 16g protein
- 2g total fat
- 0.5g saturated fat,
- 0 trans-fat,
- 11g carbohydrates
- 34mg cholesterol
- 380mg sodium
- 1g fiber

Spicy Rigatoni With Mussels

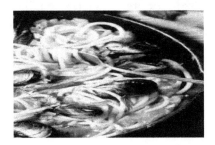

Ingredients

- 1 pound rigatoni pasta
- ½ cup dry white wine
- 2 pounds mussels, scrubbed and debearded (discard any open mussels) 2
- tablespoons extra-virgin olive oil
- 2 cloves fresh garlic, minced
- 1½ cups cherry tomatoes, halved
- 1 teaspoon red hot pepper, diced (optional)
- Salt and freshly ground pepper to taste
- 10–12 arugula leaves, chopped

Preparation

Bring water to a boil, add pasta, and cook pasta until al dente. Remove from heat, drain pasta, and return to pot, drizzling with scant amount of olive oil to keep pasta from sticking together. Set aside. In another pot over high heat, add wine and mussels. Cook until mussels open. Discard any that do not open. Remove cooked mussels from liquid. Set aside. Sieve mussel liquid, reserve liquid only. Shell mussels except for 12 mussels (to be used for garnish). In large skillet heat olive oil, add garlic, and sauté. Add tomatoes and hot pepper and sauté for a few minutes. Add shelled mussels and 3–4 teaspoons of mussel liquid and season mixture with salt and pepper to taste. Place pasta in a large pasta server, fluff noodles with a fork, and toss with garlic–mussel mixture. Scatter arugula leaves over top, garnish with unshelled mussels, and serve. Approx. 454 calories per serving

Nutritional Value

- 31g protein
- 10g total fat
- 1g saturated fat
- 0 trans fat
- 54g carbohydrates
- 44mg cholesterol
- 463mg sodium
- 8g fiber

Broiled Tuna And Tomato

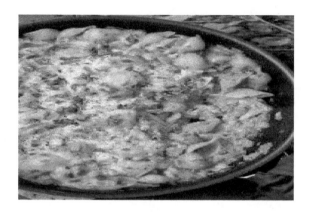

Ingredients

- 4 (3-ounce) tuna fillets
- 4 tablespoons extra-virgin olive oil
- 2 large cloves fresh garlic, minced
- 1 tablespoon chopped fresh parsley
- Salt and freshly ground pepper to taste
- 1½ teaspoons white wine vinegar
- 8 (½-inch) slices fresh tomato

Preparation

Fresh Italian parsley, chopped, for garnish. Rinse fillets, pat dry, and set aside. Combine in a covered container 2 tablespoons olive oil, garlic, parsley, and salt and pepper. Add fillets, turning to coat well. Marinate fillets at room temperature for 2 hours. In another bowl, combine remaining olive oil, vinegar, and salt and pepper, if desired. Arrange sliced tomatoes in a flat container in one layer and pour oil mixture over tomatoes; marinate at room temperature for 2 hours. Heat broiler, place tuna on grilling pan about 4 inches below heat, and broil each side of fillets for about 2–3 minutes. Arrange 2 slices of tomato on each plate; add tuna fillets to top of tomatoes and garnish with parsley. Serve while hot. Approx. 224 calories per serving

Nutritional Value

20g protein, 18g total fat, 2.8g saturated fat, 0 trans fat, 2g carbohydrates, 38mg cholesterol, 35mg sodium, 0 fiber

Salmon Cakes With Sour Cream Dill Sauce

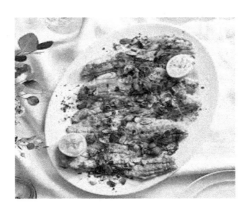

Ingredients

- 2 (14.75-ounce) cans of salmon
- 2 tablespoons extra-virgin olive oil, divided
- ¾ cup chopped scallions
- 3 cloves fresh garlic, minced
- ½ teaspoon crushed red hot pepper flakes
- 2 eggs
- ½ tablespoon lime juice
- 3 tablespoons cornstarch
- Salt and freshly ground pepper to taste
- 1 cup fat-free or low-fat sour cream (optional)
- 4 tablespoons finely chopped fresh dill (optional)

Preparation

Drain and separate salmon; set aside. In a heavy-bottomed skillet over medium-low heat, add 2 teaspoons olive oil, scallions, garlic, and hot pepper flakes. Sauté until scallions are soft, then set aside. In a bowl whisk together eggs, lime juice, cornstarch, and salt and pepper. Add egg mixture to scallion mixture and gently fold in salmon. Form salmon mixture into 8 cakes and refrigerate for about 30 minutes. Pour remaining olive oil into a large skillet over medium-low heat and add chilled salmon cakes. Slowly sauté cakes for about 2–3 minutes on each side until heated through. Mix sour cream and dill together and serve each salmon cake garnished with a tablespoon of sour cream and dill sauce, if desired. Approx. 251 calories per serving

Nutritional Value
- 24g protein
- 15g total fat
- 3g saturated fat
- 0 trans fat

Trout Almandine

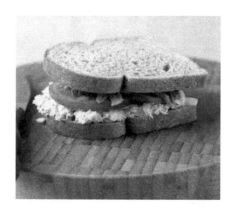

Ingredients

- 4 (4-ounce) trout fillets
- 1½ tablespoons trans fat–free canola/olive oil spread, melted
- 3 tablespoons fresh lemon juice
- ½ teaspoon dried thyme
- 1 tablespoon finely chopped white onion
- Salt to taste
- Paprika to sprinkle
- 3 tablespoons finely chopped fresh parsley
- ¼ cup sliced raw almonds
- Canola oil cooking spray
- 4 lemon wedges for garnish

Rinse fillets under cold water and pat dry with paper towels. Combine melted canola/olive oil spread, lemon juice, thyme, onion, and salt in a small mixing bowl and whisk to blend flavors. Place fillets in a single layer in an oven-safe casserole dish and pour mixture over fish. Allow mixture to get under fillets as well. Top each fillet with paprika and parsley. Bake at 375 degrees for 12–15 minutes or until fish flakes easily and is opaque in color. Turn oven to broil. Top fish with almonds and spray with a scant amount of cooking spray. Place fillets about 4 inches under broiler and broil fillets for 2–3 minutes or until almonds are lightly toasted. Remove from broiler and serve immediately with lemon wedges. Approx. 184 calories per serving

Nutritional Value
24g protein, 10g total fat, 1g saturated fat, 0 trans fat, 2g carbohydrates, 60mg cholesterol, 51mg sodium, 1g fib

Sautéed Mixed Fish Over Garlic Couscous

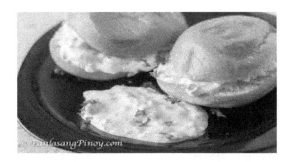

Ingredients

- 1 pound codfish, cut into 1-inch pieces
- ½ pound raw shrimp, peeled, deveined, and coarsely chopped
- ½ pound bay scallops
- 4 scallions, sliced
- ½ cup chopped fresh chives
- ½ cup chopped fresh parsley
- 3 tablespoons bread crumbs
- 1 tablespoon Dijon mustard
- 1 tablespoon light mayonnaise
- 2 eggs, beaten
- Salt and freshly ground pepper to taste
- 2 tablespoons olive oil
- Hot sauce to taste (optional)
- 2 (5.4-ounce) boxes garlic-flavored couscous

Preparation

In a large bowl, combine codfish, shrimp, scallops, scallions, chives, parsley, bread crumbs, mustard, mayonnaise, eggs, and salt and pepper to taste. Using a large spoon, mix ingredients. In a large skillet, heat olive oil over medium heat. Add fish mixture and cook, stirring often, until fish is cooked through and lightly browned. Sprinkle with hot sauce, if desired. Reduce heat to very low and cover to keep warm. Prepare couscous as per package instructions. Divide fish into 6 portions and serve over couscous. Approx. 172 calories per serving.

Nutritional Value

30g protein, 6g total fat, 0 saturated fat, 0 trans fat, 43g carbohydrates, 157mg cholesterol, 323mg sodium, 1g fiber.

Grilled Cod

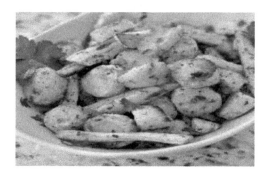

Ingredients

- 1½ pounds fresh codfish
- Olive oil cooking spray
- Salt to taste
- ¼ teaspoon freshly ground pepper
- ⅛ teaspoon garlic powder
- 2 tablespoons trans fat–free canola/olive oil spread
- 2 tablespoons freshly squeezed lemon juice
- Lemon wedges

Preparation

Heat grill to medium-high heat. Place a rimmed baking sheet on grill. Spray both sides of fish with cooking oil and sprinkle fish with salt, pepper, and garlic powder. Place fish on baking sheet and grill, turning once, until opaque (about 3–5 minutes per side depending on thickness). In a small microwavable bowl, combine canola/olive oil spread and lemon juice and melt in microwave. Drizzle fish with mixture and serve with lemon wedges. Approx. 189 calories per serving.

Nutritional Value

30g protein, 6g total fat, 2g saturated fat, 0 trans fat, 0 carbohydrates, 63mg cholesterol, 170mg sodium, 0 fiber

Peppered Fillet Of Sole

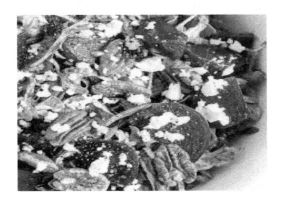

Ingredients

- 1 tablespoon olive oil
- 1 tablespoon trans fat–free canola/olive oil spread 2 cups sliced button
- mushrooms
- 1 medium shallot, finely chopped
- 4 (4-ounce) sole fillets
- 1 teaspoon lemon pepper seasoning
- 1 teaspoon paprika
- Cayenne pepper to taste
- 1 medium tomato, chopped
- 2 scallions, thinly sliced

Preparation

In a large skillet over medium heat, melt olive oil and canola/olive oil spread. Add mushrooms and shallot and sauté until soft. Place fillets over mushroom mixture. Sprinkle each fillet with lemon pepper seasoning, paprika, and cayenne. Cover skillet and cook over medium heat until fish flakes easily. Divide into 4 portions and sprinkle each serving with tomatoes and scallions. Serve while hot. Approx. 203 calories per serving

Nutritional Value

31g protein, 8g total fat, 2g saturated fat, 0 trans fat, 0 carbohydrates, 86mg
cholesterol, 158mg sodium, <0.5g

Lemon-Pepper Salmon

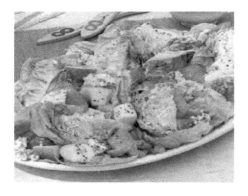

Ingredients

- Olive oil cooking spray
- 2 (4–5-ounce) salmon fillets, skinless
- Lemon pepper seasoning to taste
- A lemon, cut in wedges for garnish

Preparation

Preheat oven to 450 degrees. Lightly spray a cast-iron skillet with cooking oil and place in oven to heat. While oven is heating, rinse fillets and pat dry with paper towels. Season 1 side of each fillet with a generous amount of lemon pepper seasoning. When oven reaches desired temperature, place fillets seasoned side down on hot skillet and cook for roughly 10–15 minutes, turning once after about 6–7 minutes. Cook until fish flakes easily and serve with lemon wedges. Approx. 259 calories per serving

Nutritional Value

28g protein, 15g total fat, 3g saturated fat, 0 trans fat, 0 carbohydrates, 84mg
cholesterol, 84mg sodium, 0 fiber

Parmesan-Crusted Fish

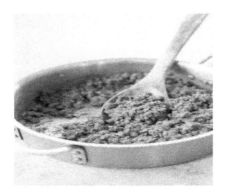

Ingredients

- Olive oil cooking spray
- ⅓ cup panko bread crumbs
- ¼ cup finely shredded Parmesan cheese
- Salt and freshly ground pepper to taste
- 4 codfish fillets (about 1–1½ pounds)
- ¼ cup melted trans fat–free canola/olive oil spread ½ tablespoon fresh garlic paste blend

Preparation

Preheat oven to 350 degrees. Lightly spray a baking sheet with cooking oil. In a large, shallow baking dish, mix together panko bread crumbs, Parmesan cheese, and salt and pepper to taste. Roll fillets in mixture to coat all sides. Blend together melted canola/olive oil spread and garlic paste in a small bowl. Place

Grilled Blackened Salmon

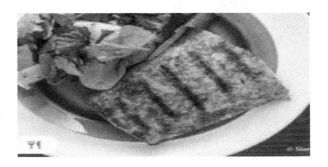

Ingredients

- A teaspoon sea salt
- A tablespoon paprika
- A teaspoon onion powder
- A teaspoon garlic powder
- A teaspoon cayenne pepper
- A teaspoon mixed pepper flakes
- Half teaspoon dried thyme
- Half teaspoon dried basil
- olive oil (⅛)
- 4 salmon fillets

Preparation

Place a dry cast-iron skillet on grill and heat to 400 degrees. Mix all seasonings together. Brush both sides of fillets with scant amount of olive oil and drench both sides in seasonings. Place fillets on hot skillet and blacken each side about 3–4 minutes or until blackened and fish flakes easily. Approx. 426 calories per serving

Nutritional Value

34g protein, 19g total fat, 0.9g saturated fat, 0 trans fat, 3g carbohydrates, 130mg cholesterol, 240mg sodium, 0.7g fiber, 0mg cholesterol, 288mg sodium, 7g fiber

Great Tuna Salad On Whole Grain Toast

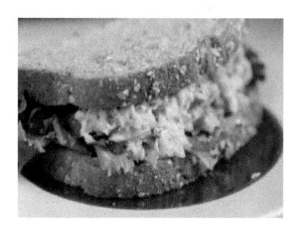

Ingredient

- 3 cans solid white albacore tuna, packed in water ¼ cup minced onion
- 8 manzanilla-stuffed green olives, sliced 1 celery rib, finely chopped
- Salt and freshly ground pepper to taste Squeeze of fresh lemon juice
- Quarter cup of light mayonnaise
- Eight slices light whole grain bread, toasted 4 crisp Romaine lettuce leaves
- 4 thick slices tomato

Preparation

Drain tuna through a strainer and press dry with paper towels. Transfer to a medium bowl and mash with a fork until finely flaked. Add onion, olive slices, celery, salt and pepper, lemon juice, and mayonnaise. Stir to blend ingredients well. Divide tuna mixture into 4 equal portions. Top each of 4 slices of toasted whole grain bread with tuna mixture, lettuce, tomato, and salt and pepper, if desired. Add top piece of toast and serve.

Nutritional value

53 calories per serving (50 calories per slice of bread) 13g protein,
0 total fat, 0 saturated fat, 0 trans fat, 20g carbohydrates, 4mg cholesterol,
378mg sodium, 4g fiber

Tuna spread

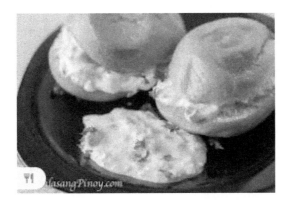

Ingredients

- 1 shallot, chopped
- 1 (8 oz.) container cream cheese spread (chives-and-onion flavor)
- 1 tsp. Italian seasoning
- 1 hard-cooked egg, finely chopped
- 1 medium tomato, coarsely chopped
- 1 (6 oz.) can tuna, drained, cut into chunks
- ½ cup pitted Kalamata olives, halved
- 1 tbsp. chopped fresh parsley
- 48 cracke

Preparation

Mix together shallot, cream cheese, and Italian seasoning in a small bowl until well blended; spread the mixture on a serving plate. Top with egg, tomato, tuna, olives, and parsley and serve with crackers.

Prosciutto Kale

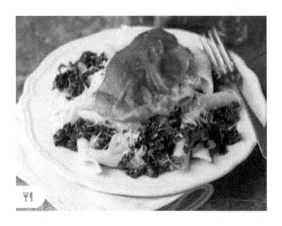

Prosciutto with kale is a winning combination. Served with trout, it's splendid.

Ingredients
- 2 Tbsp Olive Oil
- 1 Small Shallot, Chopped (About 1 Tbsp) 1 Lb/455 G Kale, Rinsed, Dried, Stemmed,
- And Coarsely Chopped
- 2 Tbsp Water
- ¼ Tsp Kosher Salt
- 2 Oz/55 G Prosciutto, Cut Into Long Threads

Preparation

In your largest, deepest frying pan, heat the oil with the shallot over medium heat. When the oil shimmers, add the kale and water. Use tongs to turn the unwieldy greens over, slowly coating them with oil to prevent the bottoms from burning. The kale will quickly wilt, making it more manageable as you continue to cook for 5 to 7 minutes. I like my kale just wilted and heated through. Add the prosciutto to just heat it once the kale is cooked to your taste.

Crispy Parsnip Rounds

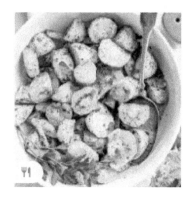

Underused and underappreciated, parsnips have a complex flavor with a sweetness that makes them perfect candidates for caramelizing. Butter, salt, and a long, slow cook are all it takes to get most of these little rounds crispy, while others remain soft.

Ingredients

- Two Bsp Butter
- A Lb/455 G Parsnips, Peeled And Thinly Sliced
- Three Sprigs Fresh Thyme
- Quarter Tsp Kosher Salt

Preparation

In a large frying pan over medium-low heat, combine the butter, parsnips, thyme, and salt. Cook, stirring frequently, for 20 to 25 minutes or until the parsnips has colored and most have become crispy. Some will blacken in spots while others may remain soft. Don't worry; they'll all be delicious

Lentils

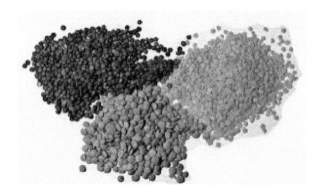

I eat lentils all the time: for breakfast with an egg on top, for lunch with a few greens, and for dinner with whatever bit of protein happens to be on my plate. Double this recipe and see what you think of a lentil obsessed existence.

Ingredients

- A Cup/220 G French Puy Lentils
- 2½ Cups/600 G Chicken Or Fish Stock
- Kosher Salt
- ¾ Cup/100 G Walnuts, Toasted Salted, And Coarsely Chopped

Preparation

In a medium saucepan, combine the lentils and chicken stock and set over medium heat. Simmer for 25 to 30 minutes, or until the lentils are tender and the liquid is absorbed. As the lentils finish cooking, watch carefully for scorching. Add some salt, stir, and taste, adding more salt as needed. Finish by sprinkling walnuts on top

Beet-Feta Salad

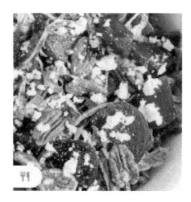

Piquant and yet sweet, this salad is a lovely complement to the clam pie. Think of it as a relish that's meant to be eaten right alongside the pie.

Ingredients

- 2 Large Red Beets , Scrubbed
- 2 Large Golden Beets, Scrubbed
- A Tbsp Olive Oil
- A Tbsp Water
- Quarter Tsp Kosher Salt
- Two Tablespoons Of Good Extra-Virgin Olive Oil
- 1 Tsp White Wine Vinegar
- Flaky Or Coarse Salt
- 3½ Oz/100 G Feta (I Like The French-Made Valbreso)

Preparation

Preheat the oven to 350°F/180°C/gas 4. Place a large sheet of foil on a baking sheet. Lay the beets in the center, sprinkle on the tbsp. of olive oil, the water, and the kosher salt. Lay a second sheet of foil on top and then crimp the edges of the two sheets together to make a tightly sealed package. Bake the beets for 40 minutes or until tender. If the skins are tough, they will slip off; if not, leave them on and eat them.

Slice the beets crosswise, and then cut each slice in half. Place the beets in a serving bowl and toss with the extravergin olive oil and vinegar. Sprinkle with a bit of flaky or coarse salt and then crumble the feta on top

Sour Apple–Bibb Lettuce Salad

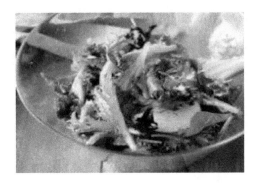

A simple salad with a bracing acidity to eat after this rich meal. It'll cleanse your palate and get you ready for a bite of cheese. Super fresh lettuce is sweet and flavorful.

Ingredients

- 1 Granny Smith Or Other Tart Apple
- 1 Tsp Fresh Lemon Juice
- 1 To 2 Heads Bibb Lettuce
- 1 Tbsp Very Good Extra-Virgin Olive Oil
- Flaky Or Coarse Salt And Black Pepper

Preparation

Peel the apple and cut it into uniform cubes the width of your pinky nail. As you work, place them in the bottom of a small bowl and toss with the lemon juice to coat. Rip the lettuce leaves into manageable pieces—maybe in quarters, depending on their size—and place them in a salad bowl. Toss the lettuce with the olive oil, a pinch of salt, and a grind of black pepper. Scatter the apple pieces on top and you're done.

Mustard Aïoli

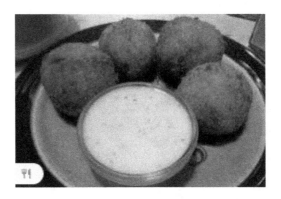

Mayonnaise is practically a food group for my southern friends. Made fresh and goosed up with a little acidity, garlic, and enough mustard to give it a ping, this version will take you through any meal.

Ingredients

- 2 Egg Yolks
- 2 Tbsp Fresh Lemon Juice
- 1 Cup/240 Ml Light Olive Oil (Not Extra-Virgin) ½ Head Garlic, Cloves Peeled And
- Minced
- 2 Tbsp Low-Acid, Grainy Mustard Such As Maille Old Style
- ½ Tsp Kosher Salt
- Black Pepper

Preparation

In a large metal bowl, beat the egg yolks vigorously using a balloon whisk. After the yolks turn light yellow, whisk in the lemon juice. Drizzle a tiny bit of olive oil into the mixture, whisking all the while. Continue adding the olive oil in a thin stream, whisking constantly, until it's all incorporated. The mixture will stiffen as the oil forms an emulsion with the egg yolks. Add the garlic, mustard, salt, and some pepper. Mix well and transfer to a pretty bowl. Refrigerate for 30 minutes before serving to give it body

Domino Potatoes

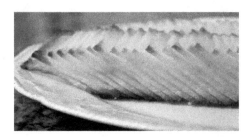

Cutting these potatoes into rectangles is worth the trouble; it's a treat to have such a stunning potato dish to bring to the table.

Ingredients
- 5 Russet Potatoes, Peeled And Set In A Bowl Of Cold Water
- 4 Tbsp/55 G Butter, Melted
- ½ Tsp Kosher Salt

Preparation

Preheat the oven to 400°F/200°C/gas 6. Cut the potatoes into rectangles by cutting off the rounded parts on each of the four sides and on each end. Beginning at one end, cut each potato into thin slices—but not so thin that the slice doesn't hold its shape. Put the slices in a bowl and toss gently with the butter and salt. Lay the potatoes in four rows in a 12-by-9-in/30.5-by-23-cm baking dish. Each row should look almost like toppled dominoes (if the dominoes were a little irregular and more square than rectangular). The four rows of potatoes should fit with just a little space between them. Bake for 40 to 50 minutes or until the edges are toasty brown—even black in spots—and the potatoes feel soft when a knife is inserted in the center.

Grapefruit-Fennel Salad

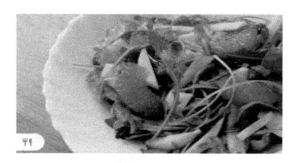

Lettuce in salad has its place, but a salad without lettuce sheds its own boundaries to become a dish in itself. This lettuce-free winter salad is one I make often: crisp, freshly toasted almond slivers with pink grapefruit and crunchy fennel. Use high-end olive oil and a Meyer lemon, if you can find one.

Ingredients

- 1 Large Fennel Bulb, Tough Outer Layer Removed, Cut Into Thin Rounds
- 3 Pink Grapefruit, Peeled
- ¾ Cup/100 G Slivered Almonds, Toasted (See Page 30)
- 2 Tbsp Very Good Extra-Virgin Olive Oil
- 1 Tbsp Fresh Lemon Juice
- ½ Tsp Kosher Salt

Preparation

Stack the fennel rounds and cut across them to make bite size chunks. Section the grapefruit, using your hands to get rid of as much of the membrane as possible, and cut into chunks. Toss the fennel, grapefruit, and ½ cup/60 g of the almonds together in a salad or large mixing bowl. Add the olive oil, lemon juice, and salt. Toss thoroughly. Finish

Cilantro Rice

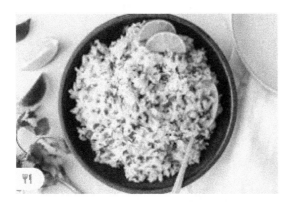

Bright, turf green, and flavorful. With this meal, I like to serve this rice at room temperature, but that's up to you.

Ingredients

- 1½ Cups/285 G Long-Grain Rice
- 1/3 Cups/315 Ml Water
- 1 Tbsp Fresh Lime Juice
- 1 Cup Coarsely Chopped Fresh Cilantro
- 4 Tbsp/55 G Butter, Melted
- ½ Tsp Kosher Salt

Preparation

Rinse the rice under cool water until the water runs clear. Drain the rice and combine it with the water in a medium pot with a tight-fitting lid. Set over medium heat and cook for 10 to 12 minutes or until the rice is tender and the water has been absorbed. In a blender combine the lime juice, cilantro, butter, and salt. Blend until smooth. Pour the cilantro mixture over the rice, mix thoroughly, and serve.

Alapeño-Cumin Butter

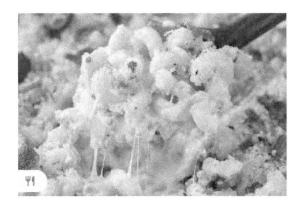

Toasted cumin mixed with jalapeño and butter. I adore these flavors and I think you will, too, when you taste them melted into your fish.

Ingredients
- 4 Tbsp/55 G Butter, At Room Temperature
- 1 Shallot, Chopped
- 2 Tbsp Cumin Seeds, Toasted (See Page 30) And Ground
- 1 Tbsp Coriander Seeds, Toasted And Ground
- 1 Jalapeño With Seeds, Minced (3 Tbsp)

Preparation
In a small bowl, mash together the butter, shallot, cumin seeds, coriander seeds, and jalapeño. Set aside.

Tomatiillo-Radish Salsa

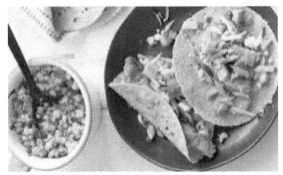

The tomatillo's citrus-scented presence is always welcome on my plate. Mixed with radishes, as here, its pretty green color and unexpected brightness carry the salsa from plain to glorious.

Ingredients

- 8 Oz/225 G Tomatillos, Peeled
- 8 French Breakfast Radishes, Trimmed
- 3 Green Onions, White And Tender Green Parts, Thinly Sliced
- ½ Cup/20 G Chopped Fresh Cilantro
- 2 Garlic Cloves, Minced
- 1 Serrano Chile, Minced, With Seeds
- 1 Tsp Kosher Salt
- 1 Tbsp Fresh Lime Juice
- 1 Tsp Cumin Seeds, Toasted (See Page 30) And Lightly Crushed

Preparation

Fill a medium bowl with cold water. Bring a medium pot filled with water to a boil and blanch the tomatillos for 1 minute, immediately transferring them to the cold water to cool. Drain, pat dry, core, and coarsely chop. Thinly slice the radishes, then cut across the slices to create small batons. In a pretty serving bowl, mix together the tomatillos, radishes, green onions, cilantro, garlic, chile, salt, lime juice, and cumin seeds. Taste for salt and heat. The salsa will mellow as it sits.

Garlic Shrimp, Red Rice, Black Beans And Roasted Pardon Chilled

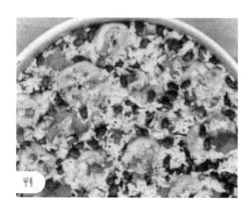

Ingredients

- Bsp Butter
- ½ Head Garlic, Peeled And Chopped
- 1½ Lb/680 G Shrimp, Peeled And Deveined
- ½ Tsp Chile Flakes
- 4 To 6 Green Onions, Thinly Sliced
- 2 Tbsp Fresh Lime Juice
- Flaky Or Coarse Salt
- ½ Cup/120 Ml Sour Cream Or Mexican Crema Red Rice (Recipe Follows) Black
- Beans (Recipe Follows) Roasted Padrón Chiles (Recipe Follows) ¼ Cup/10 G

- Chopped Fresh Cilantro

Preparation

Combine the butter and garlic over very low heat. Allow the butter to soften without getting very hot for 3 to 5 minutes. Keep the heat on low, add the shrimp and Chile flakes, and cook slowly with the garlic for 5 to 8 minutes, depending on the size of the shrimp and your heat source. When the shrimp are done—taste one—add the lime juice and adjust for salt, as needed.

Sautéed-Garlic Bok Choy

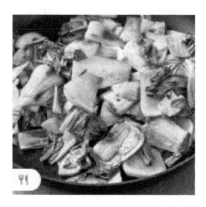

Bok choy is a mild, easy to love green. Cooked with plenty of garlic, it puts me in mind of a day in New York City's Chinatown and the irresistible bowls of greens that arrive at the table in a cloud of their own aromatic steam.

Ingredients

- 2 Tbsp Olive Oil
- ½ Head Garlic, Cloves Peeled And Sliced
- 5 Baby Or 2 Mature Heads Bok Choy, Trimmed And Coarsely Chopped
- ¼ Cup/60 Ml Water
- 1 Tbsp Soy Sauce
- Flaky Or Coarse Salt

Preparation

Put the oil in a large frying pan with a lid over medium heat. Add the garlic and let it cook for about 1 minute before adding the bok choy along with the water and soy sauce. Stir to coat the bok choy with oil and to move the garlic around. Cover and cook for 3 to 5 minutes. Remove the lid, taste, and cook for another 2 minutes or so or until the greens are tender and the pan is nearly dry. Sprinkle with a pinch of flaky or coarse salt and serve.

Goan fish curry with spicy snap peas and whole wheat rotis

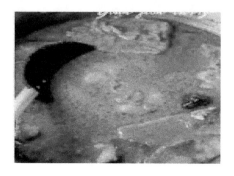

Ingredients

- 2 Tbsp Peanut Oil
- 1 Sweet Onion, Such As Vidalia, Thinly Sliced
- 2 Tbsp Yellow Mustard Seeds
- 1 Cinnamon Stick
- 1 Tsp Ground Turmeric
- ½ Tsp Garam Masala
- 1 Tbsp Kosher Salt
- 2 Serrano, Jalapeño, Or Dundicut Chiles (See Heat And Chiles, Page 30) 1 Thumblength Piece Fresh Ginger, Peeled And Cut Into Chunks
- 2 Large Tomatoes, Cored
- 2 Cups/480 Ml Water
- One 13½-Oz/400-Ml Can Unsweetened Coconut Milk, Fullfat

- 1 Lb/455 G Catfish Fillets, Or Other White,Flaky Fish, Cut Into 4 Or More Portions
- Basmati Rice (Page 186)
- Coconut Chutney (See Page 182)
- Spicy Snap Peas (Recipe Follows) Whole-Wheat Rotis (Recipe Follows)

Preparation

Heat a large dutch oven or a large, deep frying pan over medium heat. Add the peanut oil, onion, mustard seeds, cinnamon stick, turmeric, graham masala, and salt. Cook, stirring frequently, for 10 to 12 minutes or until the onion overshot and the spices are fragrant. While the onion cooks, combine the chilies, ginger, tomatoes, and water in a blender. Pulse briefly, just to chop—not purée—the chilies and ginger. It won't take long. Add the liquid to the onion mixture, along with the coconut milk, and stir. Cook, uncovered, over medium-low heat for another 10 to 12 minutes. You can set the curry aside at this point until 10 minutes before you're ready to eat. Reheat the ingredients and add the fish. Cook over medium heat for 8 to 10 minutes or until the fish is flaky. Taste for

✰ 55% OFF for BookStore NOW at $ 24,95 instead of $ 35,95! ✰

If you are looking for and love to eat fish, in this guide you will find everything you need to cook fantastic dishes and amaze your fellow travelers.

Have fun and cook with love

START IS NOW!!

Buy is NOW and let your Customers get addicted to this amazing book!